This is tough f*cking love B*tch!
It's time to get real!

This Planner Belongs To :

_____

(A Bad Ass B*tch In The Making!)

Time to Lose Them Pounds!

(Failure Is For Weak Ass B*tches!
Motto For The Next 90 Days: Don't Be A Weak Ass B*tch!)

Where The F*ck Am I At?

Chest

Arm

Waist

Hips

Thigh

WEIGHT:

LEFT ARM:

RIGHT ARM:

CHEST:

WAIST:

HIPS:

LEFT THIGH:

RIGHT THIGH:

START DATE:

How the F*ck did i get here?
NB: Be real, only Dumbass B*tches lie to themselves!
Consider big stressors in your life? Bad sh*t that's happened
to you? Your habits? Negative people or beliefs in your life
that may be holding you back?

Where The F*ck Do I Wanna Be At?

BE SPECIFIC. IT HELPS YOU!

GOAL MEASUREMENTS:

WEIGHT:	
LEFT ARM:	
RIGHT ARM:	
CHEST:	
WAIST:	
HIPS:	
LEFT THIGH:	
RIGHT THIGH:	

GOAL DATE:

How can i stop all that negative sh*t i listed from getting in my way?

Why's losing weight and getting fit important to me?

What's my diet plan to achieve my goals?

What's my fitness and exercise plan to achieve my goals?

I BELIEVE IN YOU B*TCH!

90 days to get it! X your progress...

1	2	3	4	5	6	7	8	9	10
11	12	13	14	15	16	17	18	19	20
21	22	23	24	25	26	27	28	29	30
31	32	33	34	35	36	37	38	39	40
41	42	43	44	45	46	47	48	49	50
51	52	53	54	55	56	57	58	59	60
61	62	63	64	65	66	67	68	69	70
71	72	73	74	75	76	77	78	79	80
81	82	83	84	85	86	87	88	89	90

Ok, B*tch, you got my attention!

30

Yes, B*tch, you on your way!

60

Officially, a Bad Ass B*tch!

90

Day 1 B*tch, let's go!

DATE:

ACTIVITY:	SETS/REPS/DISTANCE/TIME:	CALORIES BURNED? GOAL ACHIEVED?

WATER INTAKE:		SUPPLEMENTS?			
FOOD/TIME/AMOUNT		PROT.	FAT.	CARBS.	CAL.
TOTAL:					

HOW I FELT?/GOALS FOR TOMORROW?   SLEEP:

DATE:

ACTIVITY:	SETS/REPS/DISTANCE/TIME:	CALORIES BURNED? GOAL ACHIEVED?

WATER INTAKE:	SUPPLEMENTS?			
FOOD/TIME/AMOUNT	PROT.	FAT.	CARBS.	CAL.
TOTAL:				

HOW I FELT?/GOALS FOR TOMORROW?   **SLEEP:**

Time to throw all your f*cks out the door today and go get it!

DATE:

ACTIVITY:	SETS/REPS/DISTANCE/TIME:	CALORIES BURNED? GOAL ACHIEVED?

WATER INTAKE: **SUPPLEMENTS?**

FOOD/TIME/AMOUNT	PROT.	FAT.	CARBS.	CAL.
TOTAL:				

HOW I FELT?/GOALS FOR TOMORROW?   **SLEEP:**

Don't cry B*tch, YOU want this!

DATE:

ACTIVITY:	SETS/REPS/DISTANCE/TIME:	CALORIES BURNED? GOAL ACHIEVED?

WATER INTAKE:	SUPPLEMENTS?			
FOOD/TIME/AMOUNT	PROT.	FAT.	CARBS.	CAL.
TOTAL:				

HOW I FELT?/GOALS FOR TOMORROW?   **SLEEP:**

DATE:

ACTIVITY:	SETS/REPS/DISTANCE/TIME:	CALORIES BURNED? GOAL ACHIEVED?

WATER INTAKE: **SUPPLEMENTS?**

FOOD/TIME/AMOUNT	PROT.	FAT.	CARBS.	CAL.
TOTAL:				

HOW I FELT?/GOALS FOR TOMORROW?   **SLEEP:**

DATE:

ACTIVITY:	SETS/REPS/DISTANCE/TIME:	CALORIES BURNED? GOAL ACHIEVED?

WATER INTAKE: | **SUPPLEMENTS?**

FOOD/TIME/AMOUNT	PROT.	FAT.	CARBS.	CAL.
TOTAL:				

HOW I FELT?/GOALS FOR TOMORROW?   **SLEEP:**

I'm disrespectful as f*ck?! Look in the mirror and tell me you can't Do Better? Be Better? Feel better? I'm for you. Always remember that!

DATE:

ACTIVITY:	SETS/REPS/DISTANCE/TIME:	CALORIES BURNED? GOAL ACHIEVED?

WATER INTAKE: **SUPPLEMENTS?**

FOOD/TIME/AMOUNT	PROT.	FAT.	CARBS.	CAL.
TOTAL:				

HOW I FELT?/GOALS FOR TOMORROW?   **SLEEP:**

Oh Yeah, Bring It On!

DATE:

ACTIVITY:	SETS/REPS/DISTANCE/TIME:	CALORIES BURNED? GOAL ACHIEVED?

WATER INTAKE:	SUPPLEMENTS?			
FOOD/TIME/AMOUNT	PROT.	FAT.	CARBS.	CAL.
TOTAL:				

HOW I FELT?/GOALS FOR TOMORROW?   **SLEEP:**

DATE:

ACTIVITY:	SETS/REPS/DISTANCE/TIME:	CALORIES BURNED? GOAL ACHIEVED?

WATER INTAKE:		SUPPLEMENTS?			
FOOD/TIME/AMOUNT		PROT.	FAT.	CARBS.	CAL.
TOTAL:					

HOW I FELT?/GOALS FOR TOMORROW?   SLEEP:

DATE:

ACTIVITY:	SETS/REPS/DISTANCE/TIME:	CALORIES BURNED? GOAL ACHIEVED?

WATER INTAKE: 🥤 🥤 🥤 🥤 🥤 🥤 🥤   SUPPLEMENTS?

FOOD/TIME/AMOUNT	PROT.	FAT.	CARBS.	CAL.
TOTAL:				

HOW I FELT?/GOALS FOR TOMORROW?   SLEEP:

No one said it'd be easy, but at the end it's gonna feel SOOOOO GOOOOD!

DATE:

ACTIVITY:	SETS/REPS/DISTANCE/TIME:	CALORIES BURNED? GOAL ACHIEVED?

WATER INTAKE:	SUPPLEMENTS?			
FOOD/TIME/AMOUNT	PROT.	FAT.	CARBS.	CAL.
TOTAL:				

HOW I FELT?/GOALS FOR TOMORROW?   SLEEP:

GET YOUR BUTT UP AND AT IT!

DATE:

ACTIVITY:	SETS/REPS/DISTANCE/TIME:	CALORIES BURNED? GOAL ACHIEVED?

WATER INTAKE:									SUPPLEMENTS?			
FOOD/TIME/AMOUNT									PROT.	FAT.	CARBS.	CAL.
TOTAL:			

HOW I FELT?/GOALS FOR TOMORROW?   SLEEP:

DATE:

ACTIVITY:	SETS/REPS/DISTANCE/TIME:	CALORIES BURNED? GOAL ACHIEVED?

WATER INTAKE:	SUPPLEMENTS?		

FOOD/TIME/AMOUNT	PROT.	FAT.	CARBS.	CAL.
TOTAL:				

HOW I FELT?/GOALS FOR TOMORROW?   **SLEEP:**

DATE:

ACTIVITY:	SETS/REPS/DISTANCE/TIME:	CALORIES BURNED? GOAL ACHIEVED?

WATER INTAKE: SUPPLEMENTS?

FOOD/TIME/AMOUNT	PROT.	FAT.	CARBS.	CAL.
TOTAL:				

HOW I FELT?/GOALS FOR TOMORROW?   SLEEP:

Freestyle battle against yourself B*tch and then tell me you don't wanna carry on!

DATE:

ACTIVITY:	SETS/REPS/DISTANCE/TIME:	CALORIES BURNED? GOAL ACHIEVED?

WATER INTAKE: | **SUPPLEMENTS?**

FOOD/TIME/AMOUNT	PROT.	FAT.	CARBS.	CAL.
TOTAL:				

HOW I FELT?/GOALS FOR TOMORROW?   **SLEEP:**

This sh*t's important. Are you making it a priority?

DATE:

ACTIVITY:	SETS/REPS/DISTANCE/TIME:	CALORIES BURNED? GOAL ACHIEVED?

WATER INTAKE:	SUPPLEMENTS?			
FOOD/TIME/AMOUNT	PROT.	FAT.	CARBS.	CAL.
TOTAL:				

HOW I FELT?/GOALS FOR TOMORROW?   SLEEP:

DATE:

ACTIVITY:	SETS/REPS/DISTANCE/TIME:	CALORIES BURNED? GOAL ACHIEVED?

WATER INTAKE:	SUPPLEMENTS?

FOOD/TIME/AMOUNT	PROT.	FAT.	CARBS.	CAL.
TOTAL:				

HOW I FELT?/GOALS FOR TOMORROW?   **SLEEP:**

DATE:

ACTIVITY:	SETS/REPS/DISTANCE/TIME:	CALORIES BURNED? GOAL ACHIEVED?

WATER INTAKE:	SUPPLEMENTS?			
FOOD/TIME/AMOUNT	PROT.	FAT.	CARBS.	CAL.
TOTAL:				

HOW I FELT?/GOALS FOR TOMORROW?   **SLEEP:**

Be good to your body B*tch! It's ride or die for you! Love it! Respect It!

DATE:

ACTIVITY:	SETS/REPS/DISTANCE/TIME:	CALORIES BURNED? GOAL ACHIEVED?

WATER INTAKE: **SUPPLEMENTS?**

FOOD/TIME/AMOUNT	PROT.	FAT.	CARBS.	CAL.
TOTAL:				

HOW I FELT?/GOALS FOR TOMORROW?   **SLEEP:**

That's right, F*ck good enough!... be the BEST YOU CAN BE!

DATE:

ACTIVITY:	SETS/REPS/DISTANCE/TIME:	CALORIES BURNED? GOAL ACHIEVED?

WATER INTAKE: SUPPLEMENTS?

FOOD/TIME/AMOUNT	PROT.	FAT.	CARBS.	CAL.
TOTAL:				

HOW I FELT?/GOALS FOR TOMORROW?   SLEEP:

DATE:

ACTIVITY:	SETS/REPS/DISTANCE/TIME:	CALORIES BURNED? GOAL ACHIEVED?

WATER INTAKE: **SUPPLEMENTS?**

FOOD/TIME/AMOUNT	PROT.	FAT.	CARBS.	CAL.
TOTAL:				

HOW I FELT?/GOALS FOR TOMORROW?   **SLEEP:**

DATE:

ACTIVITY:	SETS/REPS/DISTANCE/TIME:	CALORIES BURNED? GOAL ACHIEVED?

WATER INTAKE:	SUPPLEMENTS?

FOOD/TIME/AMOUNT	PROT.	FAT.	CARBS.	CAL.
TOTAL:				

HOW I FELT?/GOALS FOR TOMORROW?   SLEEP:

Carpe Diem B*tch! Memento Mori! If you don't know what they mean, google it B*tch and NOW TELL ME NO.

DATE:

ACTIVITY:	SETS/REPS/DISTANCE/TIME:	CALORIES BURNED? GOAL ACHIEVED?

WATER INTAKE: ☐ ☐ ☐ ☐ ☐ ☐ ☐ ☐ | **SUPPLEMENTS?**

FOOD/TIME/AMOUNT	PROT.	FAT.	CARBS.	CAL.
TOTAL:				

HOW I FELT?/GOALS FOR TOMORROW?   **SLEEP:**

Oh Yeah, You On It Now!

DATE:

ACTIVITY:	SETS/REPS/DISTANCE/TIME:	CALORIES BURNED? GOAL ACHIEVED?

WATER INTAKE:			SUPPLEMENTS?			

FOOD/TIME/AMOUNT	PROT.	FAT.	CARBS.	CAL.
TOTAL:				

HOW I FELT?/GOALS FOR TOMORROW?   SLEEP:

DATE:

ACTIVITY:	SETS/REPS/DISTANCE/TIME:	CALORIES BURNED? GOAL ACHIEVED?

WATER INTAKE: **SUPPLEMENTS?**

FOOD/TIME/AMOUNT	PROT.	FAT.	CARBS.	CAL.
TOTAL:				

HOW I FELT?/GOALS FOR TOMORROW?　　　　　**SLEEP:**

DATE:

ACTIVITY:	SETS/REPS/DISTANCE/TIME:	CALORIES BURNED? GOAL ACHIEVED?

WATER INTAKE:	SUPPLEMENTS?			
FOOD/TIME/AMOUNT	PROT.	FAT.	CARBS.	CAL.
TOTAL:				

HOW I FELT?/GOALS FOR TOMORROW?   **SLEEP:**

What You Got For Me Today? Actually, F*ck that! What you got FOR YOU?!

DATE:

ACTIVITY:	SETS/REPS/DISTANCE/TIME:	CALORIES BURNED? GOAL ACHIEVED?

WATER INTAKE: ☐ ☐ ☐ ☐ ☐ ☐ ☐ ☐   SUPPLEMENTS?

FOOD/TIME/AMOUNT	PROT.	FAT.	CARBS.	CAL.
TOTAL:				

HOW I FELT?/GOALS FOR TOMORROW?   SLEEP:

You can't win if you not playing the game. Now go get it!

DATE:

ACTIVITY:	SETS/REPS/DISTANCE/TIME:	CALORIES BURNED? GOAL ACHIEVED?

WATER INTAKE: SUPPLEMENTS?

FOOD/TIME/AMOUNT	PROT.	FAT.	CARBS.	CAL.
TOTAL:				

HOW I FELT?/GOALS FOR TOMORROW?   SLEEP:

DATE:

ACTIVITY:	SETS/REPS/DISTANCE/TIME:	CALORIES BURNED? GOAL ACHIEVED?

WATER INTAKE: ⬜ ⬜ ⬜ ⬜ ⬜ ⬜ ⬜ ⬜	SUPPLEMENTS?			
FOOD/TIME/AMOUNT	PROT.	FAT.	CARBS.	CAL.
TOTAL:				

HOW I FELT?/GOALS FOR TOMORROW?   **SLEEP:**

DATE:

ACTIVITY:	SETS/REPS/DISTANCE/TIME:	CALORIES BURNED? GOAL ACHIEVED?

WATER INTAKE:	SUPPLEMENTS?			
FOOD/TIME/AMOUNT	PROT.	FAT.	CARBS.	CAL.
TOTAL:				

HOW I FELT?/GOALS FOR TOMORROW?   **SLEEP:**

Status Update: I see you...

MEASUREMENTS: **LOSS/GAIN**

WEIGHT:	
LEFT ARM:	
RIGHT ARM:	
CHEST:	
WAIST:	
HIPS:	
LEFT THIGH:	
RIGHT THIGH:	

30 days! YOU MADE IT! But it's early days so don't be thinkin' you the 'ish B*tch!

How was the first 30 days? Challenges? Victories?

Goals for the next 30 days?

Your Time Is Now.

DATE:

ACTIVITY:	SETS/REPS/DISTANCE/TIME:	CALORIES BURNED? GOAL ACHIEVED?

WATER INTAKE:	SUPPLEMENTS?			
FOOD/TIME/AMOUNT	PROT.	FAT.	CARBS.	CAL.
TOTAL:				

HOW I FELT?/GOALS FOR TOMORROW?   **SLEEP:**

DATE:

ACTIVITY:	SETS/REPS/DISTANCE/TIME:	CALORIES BURNED? GOAL ACHIEVED?

WATER INTAKE:	SUPPLEMENTS?			
FOOD/TIME/AMOUNT	PROT.	FAT.	CARBS.	CAL.
TOTAL:				

HOW I FELT?/GOALS FOR TOMORROW?   **SLEEP:**

DATE:

ACTIVITY:	SETS/REPS/DISTANCE/TIME:	CALORIES BURNED? GOAL ACHIEVED?

WATER INTAKE: 🥛 🥛 🥛 🥛 🥛 🥛 🥛 🥛 | **SUPPLEMENTS?**

FOOD/TIME/AMOUNT	PROT.	FAT.	CARBS.	CAL.
TOTAL:				

HOW I FELT?/GOALS FOR TOMORROW?   **SLEEP:**

Sticking to new habits can be hard. The real good stuff ALWAYS f*cking is!

DATE:

ACTIVITY:	SETS/REPS/DISTANCE/TIME:	CALORIES BURNED? GOAL ACHIEVED?

WATER INTAKE:	SUPPLEMENTS?			
FOOD/TIME/AMOUNT	PROT.	FAT.	CARBS.	CAL.
TOTAL:				

HOW I FELT?/GOALS FOR TOMORROW?   SLEEP:

F*ck the drama. Focus on achieving your goals today!

DATE:

ACTIVITY:	SETS/REPS/DISTANCE/TIME:	CALORIES BURNED? GOAL ACHIEVED?

WATER INTAKE:	SUPPLEMENTS?			
FOOD/TIME/AMOUNT	PROT.	FAT.	CARBS.	CAL.
TOTAL:				

HOW I FELT?/GOALS FOR TOMORROW?   SLEEP:

DATE:

ACTIVITY:	SETS/REPS/DISTANCE/TIME:	CALORIES BURNED? GOAL ACHIEVED?

WATER INTAKE: SUPPLEMENTS?

FOOD/TIME/AMOUNT	PROT.	FAT.	CARBS.	CAL.
TOTAL:				

HOW I FELT?/GOALS FOR TOMORROW?   SLEEP:

DATE:

ACTIVITY:	SETS/REPS/DISTANCE/TIME:	CALORIES BURNED? GOAL ACHIEVED?

WATER INTAKE:	SUPPLEMENTS?			
FOOD/TIME/AMOUNT	PROT.	FAT.	CARBS.	CAL.
TOTAL:				

HOW I FELT?/GOALS FOR TOMORROW?   **SLEEP:**

Don't be the human version of a headache B*tch and make me come for you. Go do your sh*t that needs to get done!

DATE:

ACTIVITY:	SETS/REPS/DISTANCE/TIME:	CALORIES BURNED? GOAL ACHIEVED?

WATER INTAKE: ☐ ☐ ☐ ☐ ☐ ☐ ☐ ☐   **SUPPLEMENTS?**

FOOD/TIME/AMOUNT	PROT.	FAT.	CARBS.	CAL.
TOTAL:				

HOW I FELT?/GOALS FOR TOMORROW?   **SLEEP:**

Get it! Get it!

DATE:

ACTIVITY:	SETS/REPS/DISTANCE/TIME:	CALORIES BURNED? GOAL ACHIEVED?

WATER INTAKE:	SUPPLEMENTS?			
FOOD/TIME/AMOUNT	**PROT.**	**FAT.**	**CARBS.**	**CAL.**
TOTAL:				

HOW I FELT?/GOALS FOR TOMORROW?　　　　**SLEEP:**

DATE:

ACTIVITY:	SETS/REPS/DISTANCE/TIME:	CALORIES BURNED? GOAL ACHIEVED?

WATER INTAKE:	SUPPLEMENTS?			
FOOD/TIME/AMOUNT	PROT.	FAT.	CARBS.	CAL.
TOTAL:				

HOW I FELT?/GOALS FOR TOMORROW?   **SLEEP:**

DATE:

ACTIVITY:	SETS/REPS/DISTANCE/TIME:	CALORIES BURNED? GOAL ACHIEVED?

WATER INTAKE: ⬜ ⬜ ⬜ ⬜ ⬜ ⬜ ⬜ ⬜   **SUPPLEMENTS?**

FOOD/TIME/AMOUNT	PROT.	FAT.	CARBS.	CAL.
TOTAL:				

HOW I FELT?/GOALS FOR TOMORROW?   **SLEEP:**

I know you might be tired but in your soul are you really a Tired Ass B*tch who's gonna quit?

DATE:

ACTIVITY:	SETS/REPS/DISTANCE/TIME:	CALORIES BURNED? GOAL ACHIEVED?

WATER INTAKE:	SUPPLEMENTS?		
FOOD/TIME/AMOUNT	PROT.	FAT.	CARBS.	CAL.
TOTAL:				

HOW I FELT?/GOALS FOR TOMORROW?   **SLEEP:**

YOU want this. Remember that when that little Devil voice inside is messing with you.

DATE:

ACTIVITY:	SETS/REPS/DISTANCE/TIME:	CALORIES BURNED? GOAL ACHIEVED?

WATER INTAKE:	SUPPLEMENTS?			
FOOD/TIME/AMOUNT	PROT.	FAT.	CARBS.	CAL.
TOTAL:				

HOW I FELT?/GOALS FOR TOMORROW?   **SLEEP:**

DATE:

ACTIVITY:	SETS/REPS/DISTANCE/TIME:	CALORIES BURNED? GOAL ACHIEVED?

WATER INTAKE:	SUPPLEMENTS?			
FOOD/TIME/AMOUNT	PROT.	FAT.	CARBS.	CAL.
TOTAL:				

HOW I FELT?/GOALS FOR TOMORROW?   **SLEEP:**

DATE:

ACTIVITY:	SETS/REPS/DISTANCE/TIME:	CALORIES BURNED? GOAL ACHIEVED?

WATER INTAKE:	SUPPLEMENTS?			
FOOD/TIME/AMOUNT	PROT.	FAT.	CARBS.	CAL.
TOTAL:				

HOW I FELT?/GOALS FOR TOMORROW?   **SLEEP:**

Did your mother says she's had enough when your head was halfway out her Vagina? No B*tch! She Carried On!

DATE:

ACTIVITY:	SETS/REPS/DISTANCE/TIME:	CALORIES BURNED? GOAL ACHIEVED?

WATER INTAKE:

SUPPLEMENTS?

FOOD/TIME/AMOUNT	PROT.	FAT.	CARBS.	CAL.
TOTAL:				

HOW I FELT?/GOALS FOR TOMORROW?   SLEEP:

And she might say you're "Good, just as you are"... how sweet, but come on, we both know the truth!

DATE:

ACTIVITY:	SETS/REPS/DISTANCE/TIME:	CALORIES BURNED? GOAL ACHIEVED?

WATER INTAKE:	SUPPLEMENTS?			

FOOD/TIME/AMOUNT	PROT.	FAT.	CARBS.	CAL.
TOTAL:				

HOW I FELT?/GOALS FOR TOMORROW?   SLEEP:

DATE:

ACTIVITY:	SETS/REPS/DISTANCE/TIME:	CALORIES BURNED? GOAL ACHIEVED?

WATER INTAKE:	SUPPLEMENTS?			
FOOD/TIME/AMOUNT	PROT.	FAT.	CARBS.	CAL.
TOTAL:				

HOW I FELT?/GOALS FOR TOMORROW?   **SLEEP:**

DATE:

ACTIVITY:	SETS/REPS/DISTANCE/TIME:	CALORIES BURNED? GOAL ACHIEVED?

WATER INTAKE:	SUPPLEMENTS?			
FOOD/TIME/AMOUNT	PROT.	FAT.	CARBS.	CAL.
TOTAL:				

HOW I FELT?/GOALS FOR TOMORROW?   **SLEEP:**

Sweat it up and refuel. What stats you got today?

DATE:

ACTIVITY:	SETS/REPS/DISTANCE/TIME:	CALORIES BURNED? GOAL ACHIEVED?

WATER INTAKE:	SUPPLEMENTS?			
FOOD/TIME/AMOUNT	PROT.	FAT.	CARBS.	CAL.
TOTAL:				

HOW I FELT?/GOALS FOR TOMORROW?   SLEEP:

The World is JUICY! Are you ready to take a big F*CKING BITE AND GET YOU YOURS?!

DATE:

ACTIVITY:	SETS/REPS/DISTANCE/TIME:	CALORIES BURNED? GOAL ACHIEVED?

WATER INTAKE: **SUPPLEMENTS?**

FOOD/TIME/AMOUNT	PROT.	FAT.	CARBS.	CAL.
TOTAL:				

HOW I FELT?/GOALS FOR TOMORROW?   **SLEEP:**

DATE:

ACTIVITY:	SETS/REPS/DISTANCE/TIME:	CALORIES BURNED? GOAL ACHIEVED?

WATER INTAKE:	SUPPLEMENTS?

FOOD/TIME/AMOUNT	PROT.	FAT.	CARBS.	CAL.
TOTAL:				

HOW I FELT?/GOALS FOR TOMORROW?   SLEEP:

DATE:

ACTIVITY:	SETS/REPS/DISTANCE/TIME:	CALORIES BURNED? GOAL ACHIEVED?

WATER INTAKE: SUPPLEMENTS?

FOOD/TIME/AMOUNT	PROT.	FAT.	CARBS.	CAL.
TOTAL:				

HOW I FELT?/GOALS FOR TOMORROW?   SLEEP:

You deserve better. You know this. So what's really stopping you?

DATE:

ACTIVITY:	SETS/REPS/DISTANCE/TIME:	CALORIES BURNED? GOAL ACHIEVED?

WATER INTAKE: SUPPLEMENTS?

FOOD/TIME/AMOUNT	PROT.	FAT.	CARBS.	CAL.
TOTAL:				

HOW I FELT?/GOALS FOR TOMORROW?   SLEEP:

Ah yeah, now we getting it...

DATE:

ACTIVITY:	SETS/REPS/DISTANCE/TIME:	CALORIES BURNED? GOAL ACHIEVED?

WATER INTAKE:	SUPPLEMENTS?			

FOOD/TIME/AMOUNT	PROT.	FAT.	CARBS.	CAL.
TOTAL:				

HOW I FELT?/GOALS FOR TOMORROW?   **SLEEP:**

DATE:

ACTIVITY:	SETS/REPS/DISTANCE/TIME:	CALORIES BURNED? GOAL ACHIEVED?

WATER INTAKE:		SUPPLEMENTS?			
FOOD/TIME/AMOUNT	**PROT.**	**FAT.**	**CARBS.**	**CAL.**	
TOTAL:					

HOW I FELT?/GOALS FOR TOMORROW?   **SLEEP:**

DATE:

ACTIVITY:	SETS/REPS/DISTANCE/TIME:	CALORIES BURNED? GOAL ACHIEVED?

WATER INTAKE:	SUPPLEMENTS?			
FOOD/TIME/AMOUNT	PROT.	FAT.	CARBS.	CAL.
TOTAL:				

HOW I FELT?/GOALS FOR TOMORROW?   **SLEEP:**

You might think you're the sh*t 'cause it's nearly day 60... but you ain't there yet! It's one day at a time.

DATE:

ACTIVITY:	SETS/REPS/DISTANCE/TIME:	CALORIES BURNED? GOAL ACHIEVED?

WATER INTAKE: **SUPPLEMENTS?**

FOOD/TIME/AMOUNT	PROT.	FAT.	CARBS.	CAL.
TOTAL:				

HOW I FELT?/GOALS FOR TOMORROW?   **SLEEP:**

Hmmm, my mouth is open, my head is tilted to the side... you might just have me impressed!

DATE:

ACTIVITY:	SETS/REPS/DISTANCE/TIME:	CALORIES BURNED? GOAL ACHIEVED?

WATER INTAKE: SUPPLEMENTS?

FOOD/TIME/AMOUNT	PROT.	FAT.	CARBS.	CAL.
TOTAL:				

HOW I FELT?/GOALS FOR TOMORROW?　　　　SLEEP:

DATE:

ACTIVITY:	SETS/REPS/DISTANCE/TIME:	CALORIES BURNED? GOAL ACHIEVED?

WATER INTAKE:	SUPPLEMENTS?			
FOOD/TIME/AMOUNT	PROT.	FAT.	CARBS.	CAL.
TOTAL:				

HOW I FELT?/GOALS FOR TOMORROW?   SLEEP:

Status Update: One Bad B*tch on her way!

MEASUREMENTS: **LOSS/GAIN**

WEIGHT:	
LEFT ARM:	
RIGHT ARM:	
CHEST:	
WAIST:	
HIPS:	
LEFT THIGH:	
RIGHT THIGH:	

60 days! YOU MADE IT!
Smile at yourself in the mirror today! But not for long... we still got work to do!

How was the last 30 days? Challenges? Victories?

Goals for the next 30 days?

OMG, you flying now!

DATE:

ACTIVITY:	SETS/REPS/DISTANCE/TIME:	CALORIES BURNED? GOAL ACHIEVED?

WATER INTAKE:	SUPPLEMENTS?			
FOOD/TIME/AMOUNT	PROT.	FAT.	CARBS.	CAL.
TOTAL:				

HOW I FELT?/GOALS FOR TOMORROW?   **SLEEP:**

DATE:

ACTIVITY:	SETS/REPS/DISTANCE/TIME:	CALORIES BURNED? GOAL ACHIEVED?

WATER INTAKE: ☐ ☐ ☐ ☐ ☐ ☐ ☐	SUPPLEMENTS?

FOOD/TIME/AMOUNT	PROT.	FAT.	CARBS.	CAL.
TOTAL:				

HOW I FELT?/GOALS FOR TOMORROW?   SLEEP:

Struggling? Nah, not you... you got fire in you!

DATE:

ACTIVITY:	SETS/REPS/DISTANCE/TIME:	CALORIES BURNED? GOAL ACHIEVED?

WATER INTAKE: | **SUPPLEMENTS?**

FOOD/TIME/AMOUNT	PROT.	FAT.	CARBS.	CAL.
TOTAL:				

HOW I FELT?/GOALS FOR TOMORROW?   **SLEEP:**

Don't be f*cking with me now, did you do your best today?

DATE:

ACTIVITY:	SETS/REPS/DISTANCE/TIME:	CALORIES BURNED? GOAL ACHIEVED?

WATER INTAKE:	SUPPLEMENTS?			
FOOD/TIME/AMOUNT	PROT.	FAT.	CARBS.	CAL.
TOTAL:				

HOW I FELT?/GOALS FOR TOMORROW?   **SLEEP:**

DATE:

ACTIVITY:	SETS/REPS/DISTANCE/TIME:	CALORIES BURNED? GOAL ACHIEVED?

WATER INTAKE: **SUPPLEMENTS?**

FOOD/TIME/AMOUNT	PROT.	FAT.	CARBS.	CAL.
TOTAL:				

HOW I FELT?/GOALS FOR TOMORROW?   **SLEEP:**

DATE:

ACTIVITY:	SETS/REPS/DISTANCE/TIME:	CALORIES BURNED? GOAL ACHIEVED?

WATER INTAKE:	SUPPLEMENTS?			
FOOD/TIME/AMOUNT	PROT.	FAT.	CARBS.	CAL.
TOTAL:				

HOW I FELT?/GOALS FOR TOMORROW?   **SLEEP:**

Don't tell me about what you deserve. Tell me about what you gonna earn!

DATE:

ACTIVITY:	SETS/REPS/DISTANCE/TIME:	CALORIES BURNED? GOAL ACHIEVED?

WATER INTAKE:		SUPPLEMENTS?			
FOOD/TIME/AMOUNT		PROT.	FAT.	CARBS.	CAL.
TOTAL:					

HOW I FELT?/GOALS FOR TOMORROW?   SLEEP:

Haters gonna hate so you do you. Always. Forever.

DATE:

ACTIVITY:	SETS/REPS/DISTANCE/TIME:	CALORIES BURNED? GOAL ACHIEVED?

WATER INTAKE: SUPPLEMENTS?

FOOD/TIME/AMOUNT	PROT.	FAT.	CARBS.	CAL.
TOTAL:				

HOW I FELT?/GOALS FOR TOMORROW?   SLEEP:

DATE:

ACTIVITY:	SETS/REPS/DISTANCE/TIME:	CALORIES BURNED? GOAL ACHIEVED?

WATER INTAKE:	SUPPLEMENTS?

FOOD/TIME/AMOUNT	PROT.	FAT.	CARBS.	CAL.
TOTAL:				

HOW I FELT?/GOALS FOR TOMORROW?   **SLEEP:**

DATE:

ACTIVITY:	SETS/REPS/DISTANCE/TIME:	CALORIES BURNED? GOAL ACHIEVED?

WATER INTAKE: ▯ ▯ ▯ ▯ ▯ ▯ ▯ ▯   **SUPPLEMENTS?**

FOOD/TIME/AMOUNT	PROT.	FAT.	CARBS.	CAL.
TOTAL:				

HOW I FELT?/GOALS FOR TOMORROW?   **SLEEP:**

How many F*cks are you not gonna give today?

DATE:

ACTIVITY:	SETS/REPS/DISTANCE/TIME:	CALORIES BURNED? GOAL ACHIEVED?

WATER INTAKE:	SUPPLEMENTS?			
FOOD/TIME/AMOUNT	PROT.	FAT.	CARBS.	CAL.
TOTAL:				

HOW I FELT?/GOALS FOR TOMORROW?   SLEEP:

You a take action kinda B*tch, not a fake ass shoulda-woulda-coulda B*tch!

DATE:

ACTIVITY:	SETS/REPS/DISTANCE/TIME:	CALORIES BURNED? GOAL ACHIEVED?

WATER INTAKE:	SUPPLEMENTS?			
FOOD/TIME/AMOUNT	PROT.	FAT.	CARBS.	CAL.
TOTAL:				

HOW I FELT?/GOALS FOR TOMORROW?   SLEEP:

DATE:

ACTIVITY:	SETS/REPS/DISTANCE/TIME:	CALORIES BURNED? GOAL ACHIEVED?

WATER INTAKE:	SUPPLEMENTS?		
FOOD/TIME/AMOUNT	PROT.	FAT.	CARBS.	CAL.
TOTAL:				

HOW I FELT?/GOALS FOR TOMORROW?   **SLEEP:**

DATE:

ACTIVITY:	SETS/REPS/DISTANCE/TIME:	CALORIES BURNED? GOAL ACHIEVED?

WATER INTAKE: ⌷ ⌷ ⌷ ⌷ ⌷ ⌷ ⌷ ⌷	SUPPLEMENTS?

FOOD/TIME/AMOUNT	PROT.	FAT.	CARBS.	CAL.
TOTAL:				

HOW I FELT?/GOALS FOR TOMORROW?   **SLEEP:**

It's not about skinny or fat, it's about looking and feeling damn fine, inside and out!

DATE:

ACTIVITY:	SETS/REPS/DISTANCE/TIME:	CALORIES BURNED? GOAL ACHIEVED?

WATER INTAKE:	SUPPLEMENTS?			
FOOD/TIME/AMOUNT	PROT.	FAT.	CARBS.	CAL.
TOTAL:				

HOW I FELT?/GOALS FOR TOMORROW?   **SLEEP:**

Remember yourself as a little girl. What do you want for that little girl? SHE'S RELYING ON YOU B*TCH!

DATE:

ACTIVITY:	SETS/REPS/DISTANCE/TIME:	CALORIES BURNED? GOAL ACHIEVED?

WATER INTAKE: ▯ ▯ ▯ ▯ ▯ ▯ ▯ ▯   SUPPLEMENTS?

FOOD/TIME/AMOUNT	PROT.	FAT.	CARBS.	CAL.
TOTAL:				

HOW I FELT?/GOALS FOR TOMORROW?   SLEEP:

DATE:

ACTIVITY:	SETS/REPS/DISTANCE/TIME:	CALORIES BURNED? GOAL ACHIEVED?

WATER INTAKE:	SUPPLEMENTS?			
FOOD/TIME/AMOUNT	PROT.	FAT.	CARBS.	CAL.
TOTAL:				

HOW I FELT?/GOALS FOR TOMORROW?   **SLEEP:**

DATE:

ACTIVITY:	SETS/REPS/DISTANCE/TIME:	CALORIES BURNED? GOAL ACHIEVED?

WATER INTAKE: ⬜⬜⬜⬜⬜⬜⬜⬜ **SUPPLEMENTS?**

FOOD/TIME/AMOUNT	PROT.	FAT.	CARBS.	CAL.
TOTAL:				

HOW I FELT?/GOALS FOR TOMORROW?   **SLEEP:**

Roll your eyes at me all you want but i slid out the way cause thats how i roll and now there you are in the mirror.

DATE:

ACTIVITY:	SETS/REPS/DISTANCE/TIME:	CALORIES BURNED? GOAL ACHIEVED?

WATER INTAKE:	SUPPLEMENTS?

FOOD/TIME/AMOUNT	PROT.	FAT.	CARBS.	CAL.
TOTAL:				

HOW I FELT?/GOALS FOR TOMORROW?   **SLEEP:**

Shake yo bad ass, we getting there right now ain't we B*tch!

DATE:

ACTIVITY:	SETS/REPS/DISTANCE/TIME:	CALORIES BURNED? GOAL ACHIEVED?

WATER INTAKE:		SUPPLEMENTS?			
FOOD/TIME/AMOUNT		PROT.	FAT.	CARBS.	CAL.
TOTAL:					

HOW I FELT?/GOALS FOR TOMORROW?   SLEEP:

DATE:

ACTIVITY:	SETS/REPS/DISTANCE/TIME:	CALORIES BURNED? GOAL ACHIEVED?

WATER INTAKE:	SUPPLEMENTS?			

FOOD/TIME/AMOUNT	PROT.	FAT.	CARBS.	CAL.
TOTAL:				

HOW I FELT?/GOALS FOR TOMORROW?   **SLEEP:**

DATE:

ACTIVITY:	SETS/REPS/DISTANCE/TIME:	CALORIES BURNED? GOAL ACHIEVED?

WATER INTAKE:	SUPPLEMENTS?			
FOOD/TIME/AMOUNT	**PROT.**	**FAT.**	**CARBS.**	**CAL.**
TOTAL:				

HOW I FELT?/GOALS FOR TOMORROW?   **SLEEP:**

We heading for some EPIC SH*T!

DATE:

ACTIVITY:	SETS/REPS/DISTANCE/TIME:	CALORIES BURNED? GOAL ACHIEVED?

WATER INTAKE: SUPPLEMENTS?

FOOD/TIME/AMOUNT	PROT.	FAT.	CARBS.	CAL.
TOTAL:				

HOW I FELT?/GOALS FOR TOMORROW?   SLEEP:

Dance like no one is watching! You're on your way...

DATE:

ACTIVITY:	SETS/REPS/DISTANCE/TIME:	CALORIES BURNED? GOAL ACHIEVED?

WATER INTAKE:	SUPPLEMENTS?			
FOOD/TIME/AMOUNT	PROT.	FAT.	CARBS.	CAL.
TOTAL:				

HOW I FELT?/GOALS FOR TOMORROW?   SLEEP:

DATE:

ACTIVITY:	SETS/REPS/DISTANCE/TIME:	CALORIES BURNED? GOAL ACHIEVED?

WATER INTAKE:		SUPPLEMENTS?			
FOOD/TIME/AMOUNT		PROT.	FAT.	CARBS.	CAL.
TOTAL:					

HOW I FELT?/GOALS FOR TOMORROW?   **SLEEP:**

DATE:

ACTIVITY:	SETS/REPS/DISTANCE/TIME:	CALORIES BURNED? GOAL ACHIEVED?

WATER INTAKE: ☐ ☐ ☐ ☐ ☐ ☐ ☐ **SUPPLEMENTS?**

FOOD/TIME/AMOUNT	PROT.	FAT.	CARBS.	CAL.
TOTAL:				

HOW I FELT?/GOALS FOR TOMORROW?   **SLEEP:**

F*ck me! I'm gonna sit the f*ck down or jump the f*ck up! I'm getting excited at how far you've come!

DATE:

ACTIVITY:	SETS/REPS/DISTANCE/TIME:	CALORIES BURNED? GOAL ACHIEVED?

WATER INTAKE: ☐ ☐ ☐ ☐ ☐ ☐ ☐ ☐   SUPPLEMENTS?

FOOD/TIME/AMOUNT	PROT.	FAT.	CARBS.	CAL.
TOTAL:				

HOW I FELT?/GOALS FOR TOMORROW?   SLEEP:

B*tch you SO close to Graduation!

DATE:

ACTIVITY:	SETS/REPS/DISTANCE/TIME:	CALORIES BURNED? GOAL ACHIEVED?

WATER INTAKE: **SUPPLEMENTS?**

FOOD/TIME/AMOUNT	PROT.	FAT.	CARBS.	CAL.
TOTAL:				

HOW I FELT?/GOALS FOR TOMORROW?　　　　**SLEEP:**

DATE:

ACTIVITY:	SETS/REPS/DISTANCE/TIME:	CALORIES BURNED? GOAL ACHIEVED?

WATER INTAKE:	SUPPLEMENTS?			
FOOD/TIME/AMOUNT	PROT.	FAT.	CARBS.	CAL.
TOTAL:				

HOW I FELT?/GOALS FOR TOMORROW?   **SLEEP:**

DATE:

ACTIVITY:	SETS/REPS/DISTANCE/TIME:	CALORIES BURNED? GOAL ACHIEVED?

WATER INTAKE: 🥛 🥛 🥛 🥛 🥛 🥛 🥛 🥛   **SUPPLEMENTS?**

FOOD/TIME/AMOUNT	PROT.	FAT.	CARBS.	CAL.
TOTAL:				

HOW I FELT?/GOALS FOR TOMORROW?   **SLEEP:**

Status Update: Officially one Bad Ass B*tch!

MEASUREMENTS: **LOSS/GAIN**

WEIGHT:
LEFT ARM:
RIGHT ARM:
CHEST:
WAIST:
HIPS:
LEFT THIGH:
RIGHT THIGH:

90 days! YOU F*CKING MADE IT! (THE JOURNEY IS THE GOAL!)

How was the last 30 days? Challenges? Victories?

YOU STUCK WITH THE JOURNEY! WHETHER YOU ACHIEVED YOUR SPECIFIC GOAL OR NOT (WE ALL KNOW CRAZY SH*T HAPPENS SOMETIMES,RIGHT?), HERE YOU ARE, OFFICIALLY A BAD ASS B*TCH! WHO DOESN'T QUIT AND IS READY FOR THE NEXT 90! GO GET IT!

Let's Assess How Motherf*cking Badass You Are!

Old B*tch Weight/ Fitness Level VS New BAD ASS B*TCH levels?

Did you achieve what you set out to do? Explain why or why not?

What was harder then you thought? And what steps can you take to prepare for that over the next 90 days?

Always Remember, You're F*cking Beautiful!...

Goals for your next 90 days:

Write 5 positive things about your body:

☆

☆

☆

☆

☆

... and anyone whose ever made you doubt that fact is simply a Dumb Ass B*tch! and we don't need Dumb B*tches in our lives!

Sh*t I Should Remember:

Remember to keep tracking your fitness and diet to stay accountable. Every little step you take helps you to see how far you've come and make progress!

I hope this diet and fitness planner has made your journey just that little bit easier and more light hearted.
This diet and fitness stuff can be damned hard and confusing!

If you enjoyed it, please take a moment to leave a review on the website and let me know if you'd like a second edition with some more tough love! :)

And please keep an eye out for some of our other fun planners and journals soon to be published. They will be listed under our author name :
"Funny Hunni Press"

Stay Motivated You Bad Ass B*tch!